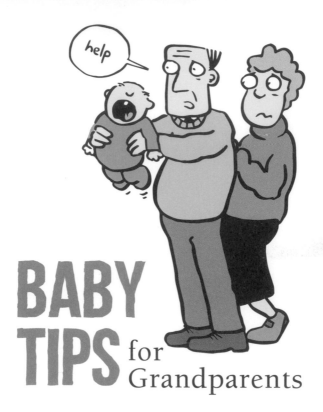

# BABY
# TIPS for
## Grandparents

**SIMON BRETT**

Illustrations by Alex Hallatt

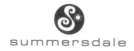

summersdale

BABY TIPS FOR GRANDPARENTS

First published in 2006
Second edition published in 2012

This edition copyright © Simon Brett, 2017

Illustrations by Alex Hallatt

Summersdale Publishers Ltd
46 West Street
Chichester
West Sussex
PO19 1RP
UK

www.summersdale.com

Printed and bound in China

ISBN: 978-1-78685-046-1

Substantial discounts on bulk quantities of Summersdale books are available to corporations, professional associations and other organisations. For details contact general enquiries: telephone: +44 (0) 1243 771107, fax: +44 (0) 1243 786300 or email: enquiries@summersdale.com.

TO.....................................

FROM................................

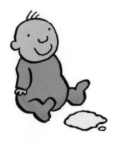

# CONTENTS

Introduction..............................6

Rocking the Cradle.....................7

General Rules...........................36

Family Occasions....................62

Nursery Rhymes......................85

# INTRODUCTION

You may think being a grandparent is easy, that all you have to do is sit back and enjoy watching the development of another generation. But being a grandparent brings all kinds of new challenges. It puts new stresses on your relationship with your children, and it's also a diplomatic minefield. You'll find, in your new role, you spend a lot of time biting your tongue to avoid saying the wrong thing.

Oh yes, it's tough. How fortunate then that you have this small book of advice to guide you through the choppy waters ahead.

# ROCKING THE CRADLE

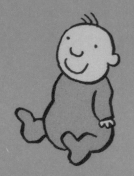

# BEFORE THE BABY'S BORN:

Try not to ask:
'Should you be doing
that in your condition?'

A grandmother-to-be should try to avoid turning into a primitive 'Wise Woman', dangling keys or needles over the bump to predict gender.

When its parents announce the name they have chosen for your grandchild, try not to wince – or, even worse, giggle.

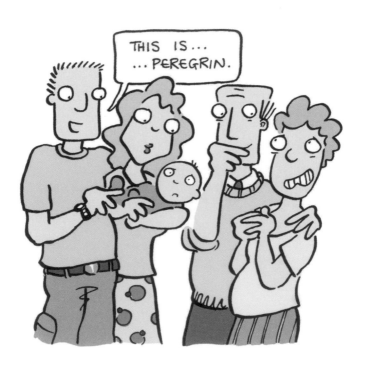

## BEFORE THE BABY'S BORN:

Don't suggest lending your books on pregnancy to the mum-to-be. Fashions in such matters have changed, and the gurus whose advice you followed have been long since discredited.

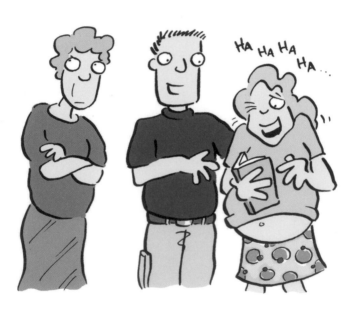

## BEFORE THE BABY'S BORN:

If you want to retain any friends, try occasionally to talk to them about something other than the impending birth.

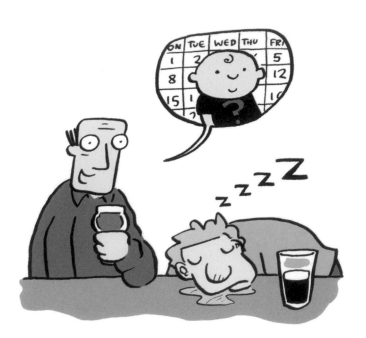

## BEFORE THE BABY'S BORN:

Don't say to first-time parents-to-be, 'You'd better make the most of your freedom now. You won't have any social life once the baby's arrived.'
It's true, but there's no point in depressing them before it happens.

# WHAT NOT TO SAY AS A GRANDPARENT:

Avoid sentences which begin, 'I always gave you...' and end, '... and you've turned out all right.'

# WHAT NOT TO SAY AS A GRANDPARENT:

Try to avoid saying,
'In our day we just
got on with it.'

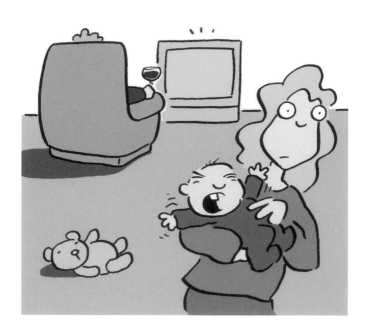

# WHAT NOT TO SAY AS A GRANDPARENT:

Or, 'The odd
non-organic vegetable
never hurt anyone.'

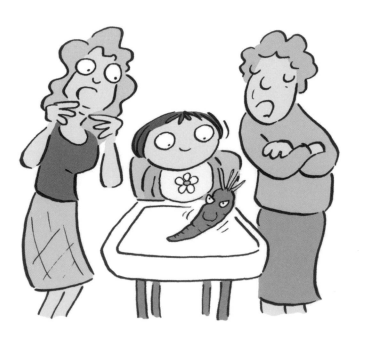

Or, 'We didn't bother with any of that nonsense when you were a baby.'

# WHAT NOT TO SAY AS A GRANDPARENT:

Never say to a first-time mum-to-be, 'You won't have time to be so fussy with the next one.' While undoubtedly true, it is not what she wants to hear.

When your grandchild
misbehaves, do not overreact
by announcing, 'I'm going
to change my will.'

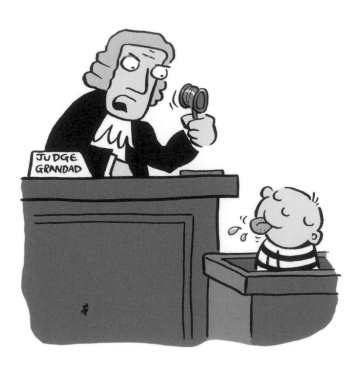

# UNAVOIDABLE CLICHÉS:

'I'm so much more
relaxed with them than
I was with my own.'

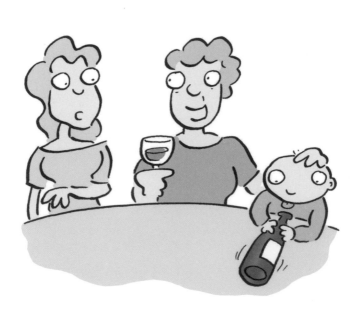

# UNAVOIDABLE CLICHÉS:

'The trouble is, these days children aren't allowed to have a childhood.'

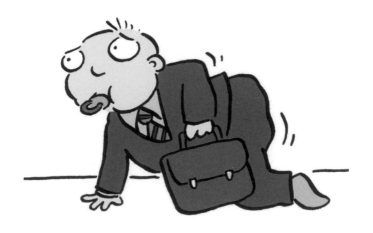

## UNAVOIDABLE CLICHÉS:

'It seems no time at all
since their parents
were that age.'

# UNAVOIDABLE CLICHÉS:

'Ooh, look, the baby's more interested in the wrapping paper than the present!'

# UNAVOIDABLE CLICHÉS:

'Well, you're
eating for two.'

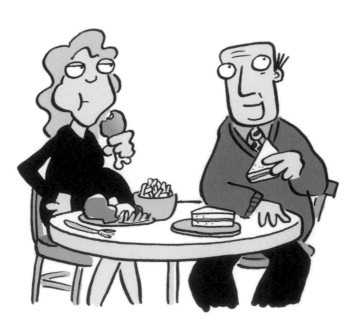

# UNAVOIDABLE CLICHÉS:

'The good thing is you can give them back at the end of the day.'

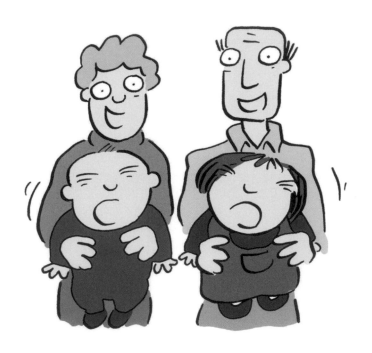

# GENERAL RULES

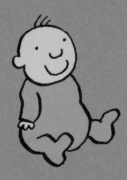

# TOP TIPS:

Never pretend you're too
young to be a grandparent.
The contradictory evidence
is there in the cot.

## TOP TIPS:

Always deny that there is any rivalry between you and the other set of grandparents. Though, of course, there is.

Do not get down on the floor
to play with your grandchild
unless you are confident you
will be able to get up again
without assistance.

Even if you've failed with
two generations, don't try
to realise your dreams
through a third.

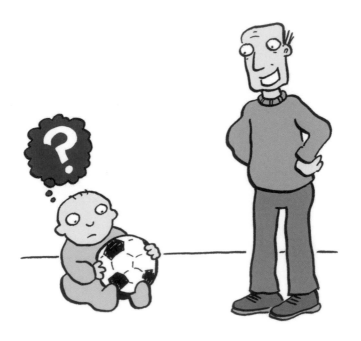

# TOP TIPS:

You will meet a lot of pathetic souls labouring under the delusion that their grandchildren are more beautiful and intelligent than yours. Ignore them – obviously they are wrong.

# WHEN YOUR GRANDCHILDREN COME TO STAY:

When its parents leave your grandchild at your house, there are bound to be tears. But you just have to pull yourself together.

## WHEN YOUR GRANDCHILDREN
## COME TO STAY:

Grandchildren will never
remember where to put
their toys, but they'll always
remember where you keep
the crisps and biscuits.

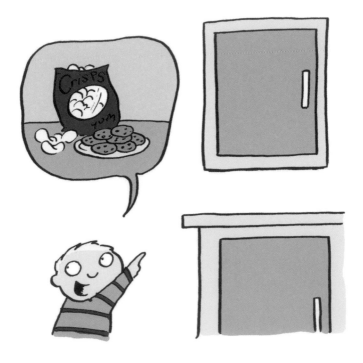

## WHEN YOUR GRANDCHILDREN COME TO STAY:

If your grandchild can crawl, remember to move breakable items out of its reach (and don't forget that a baby's reach can defy the laws of physics).

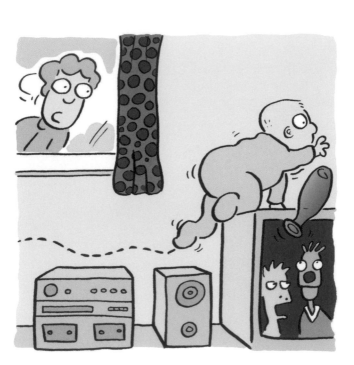

Having watched you putting DVDs in the machine's tray your grandchildren will be anxious to follow your example. Do not leave any round flat objects lying about, e.g. shortbread circles, Wagon Wheels, mini pizzas...

## WHEN YOUR GRANDCHILDREN COME TO STAY:

Early nights are very important when your grandchild comes to stay. In order to survive, you should probably be in bed by about eight.

## WHEN YOUR GRANDCHILDREN COME TO STAY:

There is an unalterable law with babies. However fast asleep they may have been when they were left in their grandparents' care, within five minutes of their parents' departure they will be screaming.

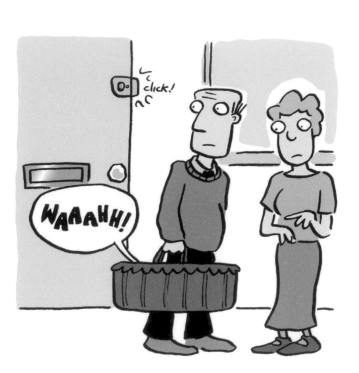

## WHEN YOUR GRANDCHILDREN COME TO STAY:

If your grandchildren come to stay with you during potty training, make sure you know the expressions that mean they want to go. This will save on your carpet-cleaning bill.

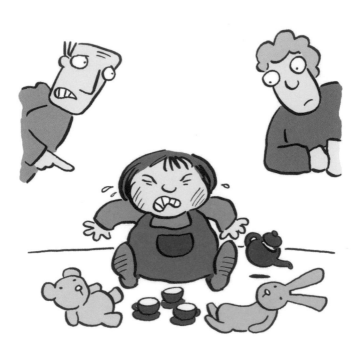

## WHEN YOUR GRANDCHILDREN COME TO STAY:

Though obviously you want all your friends and neighbours to see your grandchild, remember it is not a performing animal and may not do all its tricks to order.

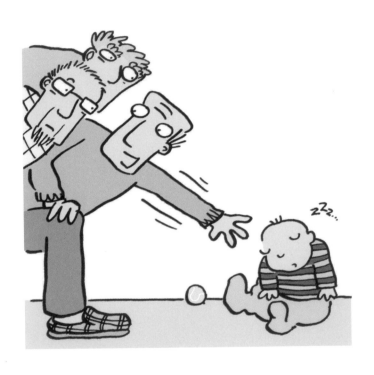

# SOME DISAPPOINTING FACTS:

Not every grandchild who does awfully good finger-painting will turn out to be the next Michelangelo.

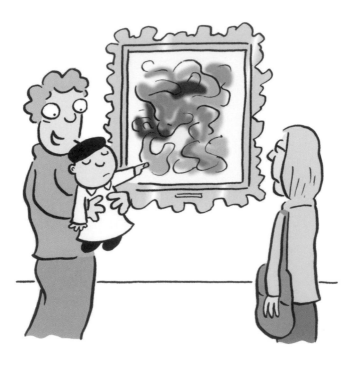

## SOME DISAPPOINTING FACTS:

Nor does every baby who looks quite cute go on to become a supermodel.

## SOME DISAPPOINTING FACTS:

Nor does every infant who is very good as an ox or ass in the school nativity play go on to become a Hollywood star.

## SOME DISAPPOINTING FACTS:

Remarkable though it
may seem, the progress of
your grandchild's potty
training is not a topic
of universal interest.

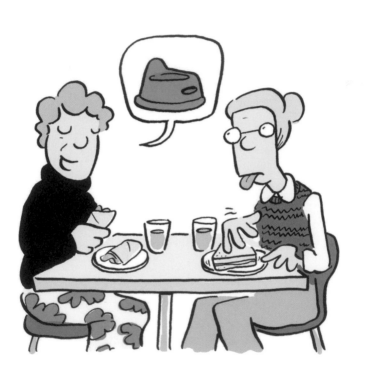

# FAMILY OCCASIONS

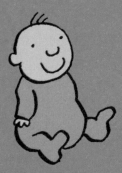

# PICTURE PERFECT:

Every now and then, allow your grandchild to do something without taking a photograph of it.

## PICTURE PERFECT:

Carry photos to show at all times. People who claim not to be as interested in your grandchildren as you are must be joking.

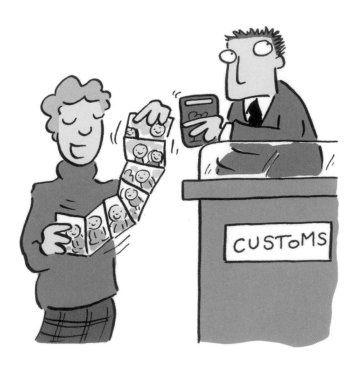

# PICTURE PERFECT:

You can spend ages with your phone poised, waiting for a smile. When you finally do press the shutter, you're almost always faced with 'not enough storage'.

## PICTURE PERFECT:

The invention of digital cameras means you don't have to get whole reels developed before you realise that your grandchild isn't smiling in any of the photos.

## PICTURE PERFECT:

Babies don't understand
the concept of pointing.
If you want them to look
in a certain direction,
make a noise.

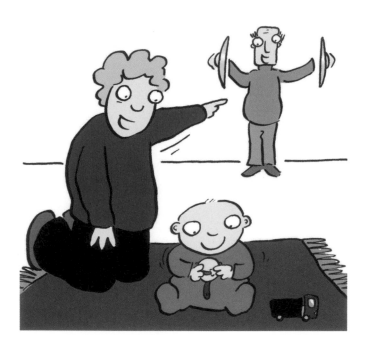

## PICTURE PERFECT:

Don't embarrass your grandchildren by knitting for them. Unsuitable garments may not last, but photographs do.

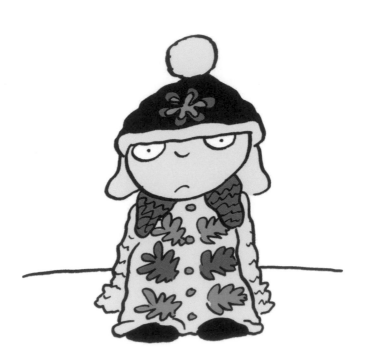

## PICTURE PERFECT:

It is the obligation of every grandparent with a mobile phone to have a picture of a grandchild as their wallpaper. This will mean that you coo every time you turn your phone on.

# PRESENTS:

If you do give a grandchild
money, do not expect to get
away with giving less the
next time. They all have
little calculators in
their brains.

## PRESENTS:

Be very careful when buying clothes for your grandchild's dolls. Giving the wrong garment can destroy your street cred forever.

## PRESENTS:

Don't give your grandchild a present every time you see them. Every now and then play hard to get.

It is astonishing the young age at which grandchildren will appreciate a gift of money.

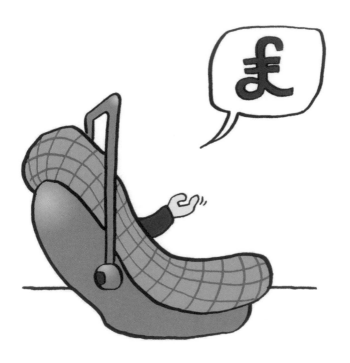

## PRESENTS:

If you give your grandchild
a present and get no thanks,
resist the instinct to ask,
'What do you say?' The child
is quite likely to reply, 'Can
I have another one?'

From a child's point of view the word 'educational' on a toy is the kiss of death.

Many parents disapprove of their children being given toy guns. No children do.

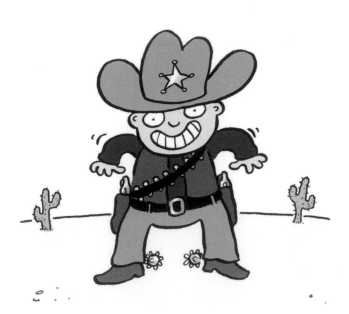

# PRESENTS:

Giving your grandchildren presents that make irritating noises is not fair on their parents... but it is quite fun.

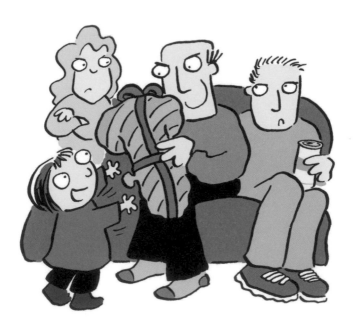

# PRESENTS:

Don't worry if your grandchild ignores your present and plays with the one given by the other set of grandparents: it plays with yours when they visit.

# NURSERY
# RHYMES

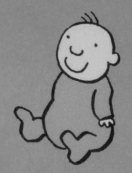

# NURSERY RHYMES:

You probably grew up with nursery rhymes, but today's children are not so likely to hear them. It is therefore important that you keep the tradition alive. Some of the old rhymes, though, may need a little updating, as in these examples...

Jack Sprat could eat no fat,
His wife could eat no lean;
And so he put her on a diet –
Obesity's obscene.

# NURSERY RHYMES:

Ding, dong, bell,
Pussy's in the well.
Who put her in?
One of those nasty
children who you must
never play with.

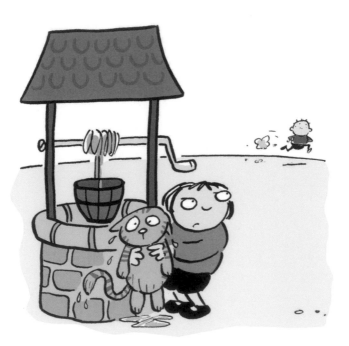

Old King Cole
Was a merry old soul,
And a merry old soul was he,
He called for his pipe,
To the pub took a stroll,
But he couldn't smoke in
The Fiddlers Three.

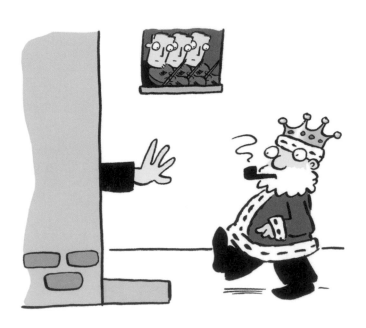

Jack and Jill went up the hill
To fetch a pail of water.
Jack fell down and broke
his crown,
And sued Jill for
negligence after.

Mary, Mary, quite contrary,
How does your garden grow?
With silver bells,
and cockle shells,
And lots of other stuff
recommended in a television
gardening show.

# A FINAL THOUGHT...

Never say, 'I'm not just a
cheap babysitting service.'
The fact is, you are.

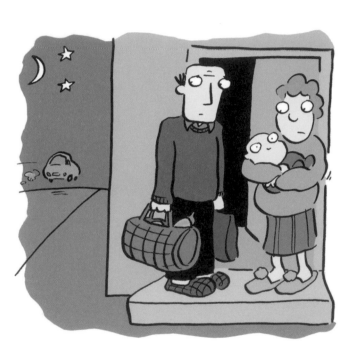

If you're interested in finding out more about our books, find us on Facebook at Summersdale Publishers and follow us on Twitter at @Summersdale.

www.summersdale.com